D1611080

C800599417

What Not to Say
to a Cancer Patient

What Not to Say to a Cancer Patient

How to talk about cancer

and create a supportive network

Paul L. Bishop

with Terri A. Boekhoff

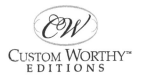

CUSTOM WORTHY™
EDITIONS

ISBN 978-1-937504-74-8 hardcover
ISBN 978-1-937504-73-1 paper
ISBN 978-1-937504-75-5 ebook

SKU CW117

Printed and bound in the United States of America.

Library of Congress Control Number: 2013948251

Dedicated to

Mike Yao, M.D., Associate Clinical Professor,
New York Medical College;

Harlan A. Pinto, M.D., Chief, Oncology Section, Palo Alto VA;

Quynh Thu Le, M.D., Professor and Department Chair,
Radiation Oncology, Stanford University;

Stanford University Hospital, Radiation Oncology Department;

and the Palo Alto VA hospital and staff

Table of Contents

Quick Reference Lists

Acknowledgments

I am one of the millions of people who have an idea which they are sure the world cannot be without, and therefore the flashes of brilliance must be memorialized in a book. My knowledge and understanding of the publishing process stopped right there, and my book would have gone no farther without the help, cajoling, mentoring, and understanding of an industry professional. There are innumerable tasks and processes that the written word has to go through before it captures the original vision, and is palatable as a book for its intended audience. My co- author, Terri Boekhoff, ably handled all of those tasks: marshalled the resources, edited the many revisions, and in general kept the book true to its original intent—the "herding of cats," if you will. I can safely say, this book would have never happened without Terri and her professionalism and persistence. My debt to her is enormous.

Graphic support was provided by Kristin Boekhoff, Gillian Kirkpatrick, and Heather Mowry. Thanks to each of you for your individual contributions.

Along the way we needed input and advice from a number of individuals who could give an honest and unstinting view of some aspect of the book. Yosaif August, Dennis McArthur, Marge Tendler, Mike Zeppegno, Valerie Pinkert, Irene Nugent, Deborah Ray, Diane Rosenblum, Ellen Bair, Heather Charles, Gayle Jensen, Sharad Samy, Larry and Jenny Crum all made thoughtful contributions. It is hard to quantify how valuable a fresh set of knowing eyes are, especially when they give you the unvarnished truth and hold you to your vision. Special thanks goes to Joel Junker and Gene Schwartz for their in-depth editorial contributions which improved and shaped the manuscript.

I have always said that my greatest asset in life has been my friends, many of whom I have had since my freshman year in high school. To be sure, in my life's journey, I have been lucky enough to meet wonderful people, and have formed a rich and deep bond with each one that like a fine wine only gets better with age. In my struggle with cancer, my friends closed ranks like the phalanxes of Greece—they never wavered, never questioned, and always stood ready to support me in any trial no matter how daunting. You know who you are. I owe you a debt that I can never repay—thank you, thank you, thank you.

One final note: When I was a sophomore in high school in 1962, I had to accompany my parents to a meeting with a naval flight surgeon. My father was a career navy pilot, a decorated veteran of WWII, who at nineteen flew off the back of the battleship *New Mexico*. He had been fighting an upper respiratory infection that he couldn't shake. I was due for a checkup so we were just combining the visits. They were unprepared when the flight surgeon told my father that he had chronic lymphatic leukemia, and they estimated he had six months to live. I was not in the room when this news was delivered, but I could see a marked difference in my parents when they emerged, and it was the first time I ever witnessed my father cry. He had no warning, like many individuals today, and he was at a loss as to how this would affect him, his wife, and five children. He was, in a word, devastated. Over the next nine years I watched my father battle leukemia, debts, depression, anxiety, work, the lack of work, and all that comes with the diagnosis. Despite heroic efforts by the staff at Bethesda Naval Hospital, my father succumbed to a gram negative infection in September of 1971 at the age of forty-nine. Today, in my situation, I understand so much more, and I marvel at his courage and fortitude in the face of daunting tasks and treatments. I miss him greatly and know that his spirit is in this book.

Paul L. Bishop

Introduction

There are few more life-altering moments than when one gets a diagnosis of cancer. Every day 4,549[1] people get this news in one form or another—that's 1,660,290 people a year. If you are fortunate enough to not be included in that number, you likely know—perhaps intimately—someone who is. If you have not yet been touched by this frightening word, at some point you may be.

I began my journey with cancer in April of 2009 when a lump was found on the left side of my neck about two inches from my collar bone during a simple, routine follow-up exam for walking pneumonia. The diagnosis turned out to be stage IV papillary thyroid cancer. When I asked them how many stages there were, I was told four. Since then I have endured two very extensive surgeries, external beam radiation for six weeks, and a variety of other treatments. One would describe me as an average white male in his sixties, divorced, and

---

[1] "Cancer Facts & Figures 2013," American Cancer Society, accessed March 21, 2013, http://www.cancer.org/acs/groups/content/@epidemiologysurveilance/documents/document/acspc-036845.pdf.

busily engaged in my life and in the treatment of my disease. I have no medical background, and a fear of needles, blood, and anything that even hints of pain. My only previous interactions with the medical community were of the normal variety save the recovery from a car accident. My chosen career has been high-end sales in both the high-tech industry with IBM and as an investment advisor to high-net-worth individuals. I love people and cherish my life.

My hope is that what I have learned through this experience, and what I have observed or learned in conversation with others battling cancer, will provide some effective coping mechanisms for those with cancer or for those closely or loosely associated with the disease who want to help. I simply want to provide some ideas and strategies that have been effective for me and for the people who support me.

To the person afflicted with cancer, this book seeks to provide strategies and resources to help you turn the people around you into a supportive network instead of a drain on your precious reserves. To those of you with someone in your life who has been diagnosed with cancer, the book seeks to help you understand the perspective of your friend or family member. Well-intentioned remarks can be frequently hurtful or inappropriate. This book illustrates what you should not say and why not to say it, and it provides you with words and actions that *are* supportive.

In the beginning of this journey, I felt like a puppet of the medical system. Someone was telling me where to go, what to do, and how high to jump. It felt like I had no control over what was happening to me, and, be clear, these people held my life in their hands. While I was happy to hand the reins over, the feeling that I had no control was pervasive. The choices that I now had to make were really important and I didn't know what I was supposed to do next. The word *patient* began to feel more and more like *victim* to me. It became clear that advocating for me was going to be important. One of the first ways in which you can do that is to decide what you will call yourself.

I choose to call myself a cancer survivor, which today is what I am. So when I am referring to the person who has been diagnosed with cancer, I may frequently use the term *survivor*. The sections of the book where I am addressing you—the cancer survivor—are identified by an "S" icon.

There are sections of this book where I speak directly to the friends and family of the person who has been diagnosed. I will frequently refer to you as *the network* because that is what you are—a supportive network. My conversations with you are intended to provide insight to the person's potential frame of mind and give suggestions for how you can best support them. These conversations are preceded by the "N" icon.

And to the amazing providers of medical care surrounding cancer, I would like to give some suggestions from the patient's point of view about how to improve your skills, monitor your presence, and provide a smoother path for those you have given your life to assist. Look for the "M" icon.

While everyone's situation is individual, I will use personal examples throughout the book. These are my experiences, and my suggestions come from that experience as well as from the observations of other cancer survivors around me and the conversations that I have had with them. I would like to emphasize that there are many successes. While there may be bad outcomes, there are also a great many good ones.

The journey all starts with a conversation.

Chapter One

Getting the News

I was standing in my sister's kitchen looking at the garden when my cell phone rang. The caller wanted me to schedule an appointment the following Tuesday with Dr. Mike Yao at the ear, nose, and throat surgical clinic at the Palo Alto VA—a teaching hospital for Stanford University. It was now Wednesday, and I did not have a good feeling about this. After the lump was discovered during that routine follow-up exam for my pneumonia, there had been a lot of lab tests and a PET scan. I inquired as to the results of those tests and was told that they were not made available to the person with whom I was speaking.

I continued to press for information. Finally, the physician on call at the VA came on the line. He reluctantly told me over the phone that he knew I had cancer of the throat, but that he just didn't know exactly how extensive it was.

The world stopped. All the outside noise, all the activity that was going to happen that afternoon or what I intended to do the next day disappeared. I became acutely aware of my time on earth, and it wasn't going to be enough. Time seemed to slow down and speed up simultaneously. Things that were enormous difficulties fifteen minutes before were no longer of consequence. Things I had taken for granted in my life—friendships, loves, familial relationships—instantly intensified. I wished that I could have deleted that phone call, but, of course, I could not.

The word cancer has a frightening impact. The word carries the connotation of fatality, suffering, and many unknowns. All of a sudden I was faced with the fact that I may have a fatal illness. Whether or not that is true, that is where your mind goes. There is no way one can be prepared to receive this news. I cycled through the emotions that most people go through—fear, anxiety, sadness. I sat for hours trying to let the information sink in. I had heard maybe half of what the doctor had told me. The power of the word when it is associated with you personally is numbing. A million things raced through my mind, all of them now cloaked with a veil of sadness. Then I realized that I would have to tell others and share this news.

For the Person Who Has Just Received the Diagnosis

Initially you are going to have more questions than answers. What is it? What do I do? How will we find out? You will likely see several specialists, have more tests, and maybe a procedure or two, then more tests. Anything that you share with others will be only partial information, and much of what you are being told you won't understand.

Here is one of the most important things I want to share with you. You have just had a horrible shock which is emotionally draining, and potentially debilitating, at least in the short run. Every person that you will tell is going to go to some extent through the shock and emotional experience that you did. They will have the same questions that you have, and they'll have some of their own. They are going to have an unguarded, visceral reaction to this news that *you* will feel. As difficult as it was to tell them your news, the wave of response back to you is even more difficult. You are trying to stay afloat emotionally. When you share the news with someone else, they go through that same struggle. You watch them engage in that struggle and you feel the pain all over again. Then they may cling to you and that can drag you down. All the professionals will tell you that they want you in the best possible frame of mind as you move through this process. You realize that you know very little about what you are telling people.

The management of your emotional health is at least as important as your physical health. As always, there is an effective way and an ineffective way to deal with the management of your emotions. So here are some suggestions for how to protect your emotional reserves.

Limit the number of people you tell initially and get their promise of confidentiality. You probably won't have much actual information for a while anyway, and you can always have a conversation later if you want to. Take an inventory of your family members, friends, or associates that are close.

When you have that initial conversation with someone you are completely drained. Now take that conversation times the number of people you have identified. You are telling the same story over and over again, and you're getting a buildup of different reactions, phone calls, emails, mail, tears, and more tears. The effect is not only cumulative, but it reinforces the fear. The draining effect of telling a lot of people diminishes your most important activities: getting lots of rest, keeping a positive attitude, and focusing on the present. The fewer people you tell in the beginning, the easier it will be for you to conserve energy and manage your emotions. Not disclosing the information right away also allows you time to get your messaging straight.

I would take a little bit of time before you tell people in order to put together a simple action plan for involving the people in your life and in your care. Identify one or two trusted people who can serve as your filter for communication and support (if you're married this will likely be your spouse). These individuals need to be emotionally stable—not controlling, not limiting—people who are genuinely interested in your well being and who are willing to do what *you* want them to do. These are the strongest, most resourceful people that you know, and they will be there no matter what. Then list the key people in your life who will need to be contacted and gather the information on how to reach them.

When you have your initial conversations with people, let them know that these one or two particular individuals that you have identified will be managing the communication around your illness. You are going to be busy handling the physical side and these individuals are taking over this responsibility to free up your time. If you are forthright and informative, people will take their cue from you. Also, let them know that they are not to disclose your information. If you feel that an individual may not honor your request, do not tell them now. You can always tell them later and chalk it up to the fog of the moment.

This is a good time for you to begin to advocate for yourself. My technique of identifying myself as a survivor and not as a victim helped me to frame my conversations with the medical professionals and to establish a positive mental attitude. I didn't get to that place immediately; I'm hoping, and recommend, that you do so more quickly.

Maintaining a positive mental attitude is essential. This is a critical element in your ongoing care; you must surround yourself with others who have a positive outlook and who are a positive influence. If you are around people who do not contribute to that, remove yourself.

As you move through the course of your treatment, you are likely to go through many tests. You may tell someone, "I'm having a test on Tuesday and I should know more by then." Well, to begin with, it's likely that you probably won't know more. Your doctor might know more but they will share with you what they think is appropriate.

Then as soon as someone knows that you are having a test, the first thing they will say is, "Call me as soon as you know something." You can see the trap here; the results may not be that good, and you may need some time to process things. Just like that first news, you may have a downward spiral and you are trying to control your own emotional situation. Now you have to go through the experience again with everyone who knows that you had the test. Each conversation reinforces what you already know and may have a depressing effect on you. And again, the result is an additional emotional drain on you from those who care most about helping you.

Be cautious about creating the expectation of additional news. There will be ample time to share important facts, and this will help you manage the access to sensitive information. Process the information first, and then decide what to share.

There are a few items that you should be especially aware of in the initial stages. Cancer has a stigma to it—there is a lot of fear, and a lot of uncertainty often based on limited or inaccurate information. Because of the reactions that people have to cancer, you may find yourself feeling isolated. People may withdraw—usually because they don't know what to do or say, but also because they are uncomfortable. In most hospitals the oncology department is in a completely separate section of the hospital. You can be physically isolated as well. While you have a new community of medical professionals and fellow members of the cancer club in your life, continue activities that you enjoy with your friends as you are able. This engagement will help to keep up a positive attitude. I had a monthly golf group that I enjoyed being around. I let them know about my situation and they let me ride with them, play a hole, skip two, and play another hole. I was exhilarated because I felt a part of the group, and I was still active.

As you are deciding who you should tell, do a quick assessment about what you want to disclose. There may be special circumstances that require this information be kept secret: work issues, sole proprietorship of a business, legal issues, and career considerations. If this is the case, be very selective in whom you confide and make it specifically clear that they are not to say anything to anyone.

I would encourage you, as soon as possible, to locate a support group for your specific type of cancer (more about this in chapter four). There are national and local groups for every type of cancer. I think you will find that these groups can be of great assistance as you put together your strategy.

The time from diagnosis to action plan will vary and may take a few weeks to a month. During this time you will likely find yourself on an emotional roller coaster. Give yourself time to reflect, and focus on what you do have control over—your mental attitude. Experiencing ups and downs is normal. While you may not be able to maintain a positive attitude all the time, I suggest you try to make it your long-term goal. You may not have control of your physical being to a degree, but

you can surround yourself with positive, hopeful thoughts
and people.

Immediate Actions for Those Recently Diagnosed

- Take time to reflect, and assess who you should tell and how much you should disclose.

- Identify one or two people that you trust to act as a filter of communication regarding your illness.

- Limit the number of people you tell initially.

- Protect your emotional interaction with others— you need to conserve your resources.

- Put together a list of people who will need to be contacted and include how to reach them.

- Develop a positive mental attitude and surround yourself with people who support that.

- Locate a support group for your specific type of cancer.

What You Can Do to Support Someone with a Diagnosis of Cancer

If a family member or friend has shared a diagnosis of cancer with you, you need to understand how important you are to them and how much they value you. You are part of an inner circle. The person who has been newly diagnosed has gone through all the emotions that you are now going through and then some. They are a bit ahead of you since they've had some time to process things. But they are still likely terrified, and they are having the same conversation that they had with you over and over again with others.

Your reaction to what they say is your first opportunity to support them. You can think of them as an emotional bank having withdrawals and deposits. You do not want to draw down their bank account; you want to be a depositor.

One of the first feelings you will likely experience is help-lessness. You want so very much to help but at this stage there is very little to do. In that vacuum people frequently say unfortunate things; they are well intentioned, but have a dev-astating effect on the person who is sharing this very personal information with you. Let's look at some of the things that people say while struggling to respond which are unintention-ally hurtful, and the impact that these statements can have on a newly diagnosed individual.

When someone responds to hearing a diagnosis of cancer with a phrase like, "Oh, my God, oh, my God," it is as if you are watching a train wreck. When you come across someone in the road with a severely broken leg you would not say, "Oh, my God, that looks horrible!" You would say, "Stay still, we'll get through this," and try to keep them calm. You would save your own reaction until later when you were alone.

I had people say to me, "That's horrible, do you have your bucket list done?" Or they said, "I had a friend who had that surgery and they lost their voice." Or they asked, "What are you going to do?" Well, I didn't know what I was going to do. Statements like that just reinforced my panic, and confirmed some of my darkest fears.

Sometimes the questions that people respond with are "Did they give you a time frame," or "How long do you have?" You have just asked me to describe the end of my life. There is a finality to this diagnosis and you have now asked me to repeat it. It's likely that I may not yet have adjusted to it or accepted it, but now I have to go through the experience of describing the end of my life all over again.

Frequently someone says, "I know how you feel." If you don't have cancer, you do not know how I feel. After we talk, you are going to move on with the normal everyday stuff of your life. You may have empathy for me and realize that I am scared, but you do not know how I feel.

When one asks, "How bad is it?" what they are emphasizing is the negative. They are asking me to relive a very painful diagnosis, and it will trigger additional questions. At this point, I know very little about my situation or the illness, and you likely don't know any more than I do. What we have are two people with no real information and a common bond of fear. That fear is debilitating, somewhat for you, and certainly for me. Pretty soon we are down in the muck and mire of really miserable emotion and pain.

When you tell me, "I know the best doctor for this," what you are suggesting to me is that my doctor is not the best. You are telling me that the person I have all my faith and confidence in is not the right person. I have hitched my wagon to this person. It's critical that I can believe in them and in their ability to help me. A statement like this undermines my confidence which creates doubt.

If you use a statement like, "I know someone with this type of cancer" which references the experience of someone else, well, you can see the potential mine field here—it might not have gone well. I don't need to hear that. It's not relevant and it's not helpful. What you are doing is taking your fear and projecting it onto me—the person who is least able to carry it right now. In truth, the research on cancer is progressing so quickly that someone even a year ago may have a very different result today.

Many people will turn to the comfort of their religious beliefs and say something like, "You need to pray." This is a very personal thing. It will either present itself as a belief or it will not. If the survivor tells you that they would like you to pray for them, it's okay to do so. But, remember your belief system is not their belief system. Even if you have gone to the same church and sat in the same pew for twenty years, things may have changed. Respond to your friend if they bring up this subject, but do not initiate a discussion in this area.

What Not to Say When You Find Out Someone Has Cancer

- Did they give you a time frame?

- How long do you have?

- How bad is it?

- What did they say to you?

- What is it?

- This is really frightening!

- This is so unfair.

- How can this be?

- I know someone who had this.

- Oh, my God!

- Do you have your bucket list done?

- What are you going to do?

- You need to pray.

- I know how you feel.

- I know the best doctor for this.

- You should get a second opinion.

- When you get the test results, call me right away.

So, what *can* you do or say that will be helpful? Start by expressing your regret as honestly and quickly as you can. Do it without emotion if possible. Let the person know that you are completely available for them, but do not say this unless you mean it. Ask them what you can do. Use short, uplifting messages, and let them talk.

One of the most powerful things you can do is to be quiet, and just listen compassionately. It sounds counter intuitive, but it is a very strong message of active listening and support. In other instances you may have the opportunity for more action, but activity does not equate to love or caring.

It may run through your mind that if you are not calling and asking how the person is, they may think that you do not care. These questions may seem like your interest in their situation shows your support, but it may have the opposite effect. Remember, many people may be doing the same thing. That may be a lot of phone calls which gives the cancer patient more to do at a time when they need to focus on what the medical team is asking of them. If they have told you about their illness, they *know* that you care. You do not need to keep checking. Waiting silently until there is a request for support may be the most helpful thing you can do.

Tell them, "If you need me, I am there for you one hundred percent, but I want to take my lead from you. When you want something, just let me know. If you don't call me, I understand that you're busy. If you do call me, I'll be there." That is real and effective comfort.

You will likely run to the internet and research everything you can on the subject. Do not bring this information back to the patient. Lots of people dragging in the newest diet trend or clinical trial will not be productive. Use the information for your own purposes, but resist the desire to share it. There is a very sophisticated team of people who are on this, professionally trained and experienced. They have not only read about the information that you have, but they actually understand it, and more.

Because you care, the most natural thing in the world is for you to want to track the patient's progress. You want to know how things are going. People commonly think of things in terms of a linear progression—diagnosis, treatment, solution. Cancer is definitely not linear. There is a lot of back and forth with varied approaches and modalities. You can imagine the burden of having to respond to every person in one's life regarding every test or procedure. As hard as it is, you need to wait until you have been given more information. In chapter four I'm going to suggest some ways that the cancer survivor can manage this information which will create a supportive network. For the time being in this early stage of knowledge, just be available when the person needs something.

What You Should Say That Is Supportive

- I'm so sorry.

- I'm here one hundred percent for you.

- When you want or need something just let me know and I'll be there.

- I'm your 911.

- I'm your soft place to fall.

- If there is something I can do, just ask.

- I'll let you tell me what you need.

- Let's be hopeful.

- Be positive.

- You seem to be doing the right things.

If you are not sure what to say, you can always listen actively.

Some Thoughts for the Medical Community about Delivering the Bad News

Before one gets a diagnosis of cancer there are clues—lab tests, activity, people calling to schedule appointments. Frequently, those little clues build anxiety. When I got the phone call to schedule an appointment with an ENT (Ear, Nose, and Throat) surgeon I knew that something was wrong; why would I need to talk to a surgeon if I didn't need surgery? But the person on the phone said that she did not have my PET scan results or have information for me. She also said that the doctor wasn't available. This was very frustrating. The appointment she was scheduling was for nearly a week away which was too long a period of time to wait. I became more and more frustrated so I pressed until I got a doctor on the phone. That's not the ideal way to get this information.

If you have this awful news to deliver, get them into your office and don't make them wait a week twisting in the wind. The information may not be as bad as they are imagining. Pick a time and say, "The doctor would like to see you tomorrow," and then deliver the news in person. Any anxiety-producing hints like, "You might want to bring someone with you," only ramps up the worry. Sometimes the scheduler will say casually, "We're just going to go over your tests." You walk in thinking it's going to be a casual chat and get hit between the eyes and you're not prepared. So don't build the appointment up, but don't dismiss it either.

How the actual news is delivered to someone is, of course, a case by case situation. It depends upon the physical information, the patient's relationship with the doctor, and the patient's personality. As the doctor delivering the news you will have to make a judgment call on what to say. There is no good way to give bad news. But there are bad ways to give bad news. Be sensitive and direct.

In my experience, most professionals who deal with cancer are very good at this part. It's difficult for you no matter how many times you have to deliver the news. In the focus groups that I've participated in with other cancer survivors, we always wanted the news delivered directly, to a person. No one wanted the diagnosis sugar coated. Now that doesn't mean we need all the gory details at the beginning. That first blast is pretty unbelievable and we need time to absorb what is happening. Inevitably, we get around to, "What do we do?" and, "Where do we go from here?" and, "What are my odds?" I suggest that you take the lead from the patient. Be direct and deliver the basic facts, but let the patient guide you with their questions. They'll let you know how much they want to know. This won't be the last conversation so all the facts don't need to come out today. You can provide the information about next steps—what tests might need to done, perhaps what some of the modalities may be, but then let them absorb the information.

Don't forget to stay positive for the patient. Instead of trying to impress upon them that this is serious (they'll get that) say, "This is going to be a difficult road, but I have a lot of success in this area and I'm going to need your cooperation." Or, you could say, "I need you to be part of the team by being engaged and involved. I want you to sign up for that." If you get their commitment early, it will engage them and get them into the team mentality. The patient needs to understand that you are a valuable resource, and that you have many patients who depend upon you. Their compliance is critical to their care, even if they don't understand why.

If an individual asks you directly, "Is this fatal?" give them the statistics. If your patient asks you, "How much time do I have?" give them the averages and also let them know that any individual may vary from the averages. Don't say, "You have this amount of time," because that quantifies and personalizes it. The truth is it's an unknown. My initial prognosis was eleven months. That was more than four years ago. So it's better to say, "Here's what our experience is, but we don't have enough information about you yet and we're just getting started here." If you are giving statistics and averages about liver cancer and they ask, "Can people live longer or shorter than that?" the answer is "certainly," which is the truth. If you stay talking about averages, you are not saying to the person this will happen to you. Averages and statistics are things that most people understand; an explanation of complex modalities is often just confusing. No matter what the survival statistic is, most people think that they will be the exception. Every cancer patient with whom I have spoken, and I have spoken to literally hundreds, believes in their uniqueness and that they will have the best possible outcome. The power and import of a physician's opinion cannot be overstated; tremendous hope resides with you.

Chapter Two

Ongoing Communication and Support

Immediately following my diagnosis of cancer in April, things began to get busy. There were a lot of tests and some of them were not much fun. I gave all of my attention to the requests of the medical team which included an ENT surgeon and an endocrinologist. They began to lay out the strategy of how to approach my illness and I just showed up. It is fair to say that I had tremendous anxiety which was lessened a great deal by the surgeon who was direct, matter of fact, and above all confident. He indicated that he had done many of these procedures. There was the preliminary task of signing documents for all the known risks in the upcoming surgery which can be pretty intimidating. In the end I just signed, what did I know? I trusted Dr. Yao; and I think that the sooner you get to a place of trust the better.

The first big step was surgery. On May 29 I had a thyroidectomy and a full left neck dissection performed. I had never had major surgery before so there was a lot that was unexpected. One of my biggest surprises was just how hard it was to get any rest in a hospital! The pain medication was really strong and kept me pretty loopy. My only initial objective was to just get out of there.

Of course, leaving the hospital didn't make the pain go away, or the fogginess, or the difficulty swallowing, or the choking. I remained tired and sore in a drug-induced daze.

Everyday mundane things were so hard—getting dressed or thinking about what to eat. What I had previously done automatically and routinely in my life, now required mental focus as my brain created new ways to perform habitual activity.

This did not stop me from attempting to reclaim my everyday life. But I should point out that seriously strong drugs alter your judgment. That may seem an obvious statement, but it certainly didn't occur to me at the time. I set up lunch meetings, and tried to get back to what felt like a normal life. But, it wasn't my normal life. I still had surgical staples in my neck closing the incision that went from behind my left ear across my collar bone and two inches to the other side of my Adam's apple. Believe it or not people actually notice that. I wasn't really helping myself by fighting the need to rest and recover. It's funny how the body will keep delivering a message until you get it. I finally gave in and started to schedule less and rest more.

In August my medical team wanted to try a radioactive iodine treatment (ablation). The purpose of this treatment is to find any remaining cancer cells that surgery may have missed. It turns out that the thyroid is a pretty important part of the body: It produces hormones that regulate your heart rate, blood pressure, and body temperature. When it's gone, you take medication that performs those functions for you for the rest of your life. In order to do this new treatment, I had to stop taking that very important medication. Every day the medication levels in my system dropped lower and I could do less and less. I felt like a wind-up toy that was winding down. At the end of the month, I could barely walk a few feet without complete exhaustion. Ironically, after going through the preparation for this treatment—taking me off of the thyroid medication—the doctors determined that the treatment would not work. They restarted my medication and in a few days I was feeling nearly normal.

There were more tests and in October the doctors began to realize that they did not get all of the cancer, and we were going to have to repeat surgery. But now, I knew what to expect. I knew what surgery would feel like, what would frighten me, and approximately how long it would take to recover. That was pretty difficult news to get. On Christmas Eve, I had a full right dissection of my neck. This time the scar went from my left ear, across my throat, over to my right ear. I repeated the recovery process, but this time around I spent a lot of time resting.

Because this was a stage IV cancer, they wanted to be aggressive. So starting on March 1st, I began six weeks of external beam radiation—five days a week, for twenty-five to thirty minutes per day. Because the radiation is directed at the head and neck area, you have to be totally immobilized which is pretty hard to do. The effects of radiation are cumulative so the treatments build in intensity. Every day is a little harder: a little more difficult to swallow, a little more difficult to speak, a little more difficult to sleep. Food lost its taste; I started drinking coffee—something I hadn't done in ten years—because it was the only thing I could taste. I discovered the brilliance of Jell-O. I became more tired, less responsive, and was really afraid. Two weeks after the treatments stopped, things slowly started turning in a positive direction. Six months later I finally felt functional. Three years later I can tell you that the effects of radiation are longer lasting than I ever would have believed. The principal effect on me was that it completely drained me. It was a full two years before I was back to about seventy-five percent of my normal energy.

Why am I sharing this? Cancer is actually many different diseases. The same type of cancer may manifest itself in different ways from one person to the next, and people can respond differently to treatment. Each person's course of illness, treatment plan, and outcome are unique. Not everyone will have the type of treatments that I did, and others will have treatments that I did not. My hope is that my experience will give you a glimpse of the need to protect your energy and your emotions if you are a cancer survivor. If you are part of the network that supports someone, I hope it's helpful for you to understand why they may withdraw, be uncommunicative, and change the previous pattern of your relationship. It's literally a fight for your life. If you recall the analogy of the survivor as a bank, you can see where multiple withdrawals will occur and the necessity of continuing to make deposits. But lots of things can make the situation easier.

Creating Support during the Treatment Stage of Your Illness

With all that you are managing, keeping track of the normal and mundane things that usually occur in your life will be hard. The importance of many of those things will slip away.

Your focus is now on survival—physical and emotional survival. You have to be able to bring your A-game as quickly as you can. You also need to be resting and doing whatever your doctor tells you to do.

For a while managing cancer can become a full-time job, and it's pretty easy to get distracted. First, a multitude of potential physical steps need to be taken. That means appointments, tests, more appointments, more tests, perhaps surgery, chemotherapy, or radiation. Part of the physical management is getting enough rest, appropriate nutrition, and doing whatever else that your medical team has advised. Second, it's essential that you pay attention to the management of your mental health—focusing on the present, maintaining a positive mental attitude, remaining calm. And third, you have a network of people who all want to know how you are, what's happening, and what they can do to help.

I suggest you establish a protocol very early with your network. This does not have to be complicated; it could be a very informal process. Let them know that as news becomes available and it is productive to release it, you will. There are lots of tests and not all of the results are good. Prepare them for the fact that even when things go well, there are ups and downs. Not all of the tests yield information that seems to inform the process so it's not very productive to report on them. One of the things that you can do is to keep the test information to yourself unless there is really something others need to know. This will eliminate the natural response on the part of your network to track your progress and check on the results. People will understand if you don't share everything.

This point is a good time to formalize your network. I suggested in the last chapter that you designate one or two people to serve as a communication filter and that you make a list of those who will need to be contacted. The people on that list are likely to be those who are pretty close to you. As you progress through treatments sharing your illness with a wider group of people may become necessary. You may have physical changes and want to explain them. There is a checklist of potential groups of people on page number 35 that may help trigger others you may also want to include. As you go through your treatment stage, instances may occur when you can use some help. This list will serve as a tool to identify individuals who might be able to help with particular tasks.

It may be useful for you, and the people helping you handle information, if you can visualize your network as a target—groups of people in each ring who may share common communication. The people in the middle are closest to you: spouse, significant other, children, parents, close friends. The next concentric ring is people that you see and interact with regularly. The next ring out is your extended network, people that you know and with whom you have a relationship, but perhaps not a particularly close one. The people from work or those related to your career may require a special type of messaging for the information that is released. The outer ring is the world at large, with which you interact—the mechanic, the doorman, the deli owner down the street.

After you have created your overall list, ranking the individuals based on where they would be placed on the target illustration may be helpful. You can direct your spokesperson to release different types of information based upon where people fall on that target.

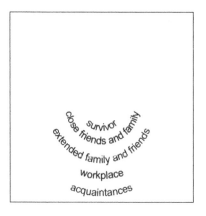

You can release different types of information based on groups.

People You May Want To Include on Your List

- Sports and fitness group: golf, cars, bowling, tennis, Pilates

- Book club

- People at work

- Hobby group: trains, quilting, photography, bird watching

- Business contacts, clients

- Religious or spiritual affiliations

- Professional organizations

- Cultural groups: theater, symphony, art, ballet

- Choir

- Boards or committees (these people share a common purpose and may be of tremendous psychological support)

The above suggestions are only to serve as a trigger for remembering people. You need to exercise discretion in who you tell and what you say, especially in the workplace.

Some individuals may decide to keep their news completely (or virtually) secret. The decision of who to tell or not tell is your prerogative. You should not feel pressured to tell anyone that you do not want to tell. If it is important to you that the information not be disclosed, be sure that you clearly convey that to anyone in whom you do confide.

If you get a call from someone saying, "What can I do?" I would tell them, "I'm on a path of recovery or treatment. I don't know what you can do at the moment, but if there is something we'll let you know. Right now my time is at a premium and I'm not interacting with people very much. It's not you; I just have to stay focused. I'm sure you understand. I have someone managing my communication to free up my time. As there is something to report, you're on that list." They will understand. Everyone who is given information should be reminded that you request that they not share it with anyone else.

It's important that you take on the responsibility for how you are going to spend your time and energy. Every interaction should be evaluated: is this conversation, event, or relationship a plus or a minus in my battle with cancer? Sooner or later you will get to the place where you discard anything that does not help you in your fight. You may have a friend who is not remaining positive and you just can't be around them right now. There may be a wedding where your attendance is strongly desired, but if you think that may be too tiring or be too difficult emotionally you will choose to pass. You are the only one who can make these decisions, but I strongly suggest you continue to advocate for yourself and let others handle their own emotions.

One of my supportive mainstays was my sister's dog, Jazzie. Pets can be a valuable part of your support system. Be sure that as you evaluate this aspect of your life you include them when they can support you. If caring for them becomes too difficult for you, find some assistance until the situation becomes manageable.

A word about hospital visits; if possible, I suggest limiting access to you while you're in the hospital. Hospitals can be draining places and you need your rest.

Don't be afraid to ask for help. Life keeps going on; the grass needs to be mowed, the kids picked up from ballet, the car taken in for servicing. It's amazing how much relief you can get by having small routine tasks handled by someone else. You have a network of people waiting to help you. A small task may make them feel less helpless.

While you have designated people to handle the communication around your illness, you do not need to stop talking to people, or participating in events if you are able. A dinner out with friends may be a wonderful diversion. Call people to just chat when you feel like it. You may find that you form new social groups because one set of friends just makes you feel cheerful. Seek companionship that is not about your illness.

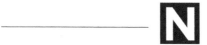

Continuing Ways to Provide Support to a Cancer Survivor

After you have received the news of someone's diagnosis of cancer and after the initial shock wears off, it's natural to want to go into action mode; doing something makes you feel helpful. You need to be aware that your desire to take action is often about you trying to process your own feelings. If you really want to be supportive, focus on what the cancer survivor expresses that they need or want and not what may make you feel better. It's okay if you want to learn more, but you should do this for your own purposes and not as something to offer up as a solution. There is a highly skilled, educated, empathetic, and patient team of professionals working on the strategy. They have all the latest research studies and years of experience at their fingertips. A really good place to find information is a support group that deals with a specific type of cancer. They usually include information for caregivers. Just remember to use this research for your own purposes.

The same cautions about what to say and not to say that were brought up in the last chapter still apply, but as you process the information regarding someone's illness and combine it with your personal life experience, some new unfortunate remarks may surface. One of the most common statements is, "I know someone who had this and it was so difficult." Well, whoever that person was, their case was unique; the other person's reflection is not in the cancer survivor's mirror. The situation of someone else has nothing to do with the person you are talking to now. Letting the cancer survivor know about situations that didn't go well is just not helpful. The truth is with cancer, whether one lives ten days or 10,000 days, everyday that one lives he or she is surviving and that is the view that one has to have.

If you have been trusted with the personal information of a diagnosis, you have an obligation to keep that information confidential. Social media tools make it so easy today for one little piece of information to become known and then be continually passed along. You do not know all of the considerations or consequences of this information if it is released in the wrong place. There may be business or career issues that are affected. The best protection for this individual is for you to say nothing. If you need to talk about it to provide some support for yourself, ask the cancer survivor if there are others that you know that have also been given the news that you can talk to and then support each other. If you find that you are really struggling with your emotions, you always have the option of seeking professional support.

In the event strong emotions make it difficult to control your feelings, be sure that you wait until you are alone to release or express them. Do not break down in front of the person with cancer. They are having a difficult enough time trying to manage their own emotions and fear. If you break down in front of them, the fear is reinforced and they now have to worry about you as well. The closer you are to them, the more likely it is that you may feel this way. Get help in the form of caregiver support groups or counseling.

You may now find that as the cancer survivor moves into a testing and treatment phase, communication with you may change. It will likely become less frequent because there is a lot for this person to do, and they are often tired. Don't take a change in the communication pattern personally. When they are feeling better, if they need something, or if they just want to talk they will let you know. They may also have a comfort level talking with someone else about a particular topic for an unknown reason—let it go.

There are some new pitfalls in conversation that can occur during the treatment and recovery process. One of these is your heightened awareness of their issue. One would think that awareness is a good thing, but it can backfire on you. If you become overly aware of what you are saying in a conversation, you may actually create an awkward moment. For example, if someone were to say to me, "I'm sorry to be such a pain in the neck," I wouldn't really give that a thought; it's a fairly common phrase. But if that sentence was followed by, "Oh my God, I'm so sorry," because they notice the scar on my neck, well, that's a different story. Now they have reminded me of my situation. Try and converse the way you always have with the person, and if you do say something that you think is unfortunate, don't call attention to it and just move on. Chances are they will not even notice.

When you are able to spend time with the cancer survivor let the survivor take the conversational lead. There are many things that are really important in their life—a career, family, business, work life, projects that are now affected by their illness. What may be important to you may not be important to them. They have narrowed their focus to only those things that are important to them. There's not a lot of room in which to add anything. A lack of focus on your life does not mean that they are not concerned about you and your issues; they just can't engage in them right now.

If you listen to them, they will tell you what is important and what it is they would like to discuss. They may bring up a familiar topic which is a diversion for them. Or, they may bring up things that they are worried about, "What about the trip to Tahiti next August?" or, "What about the twenty-fifth wedding anniversary?" Just listen supportively, but don't get into future planning. You are likely not privy to what is going to happen next and they may not be either. When you make references to how great things will be when this or that happens down the road, it may be a sharp reminder of time. For me, it often feels like I'm holding an hour glass with the sand slowly seeping out. Time has a different meaning for me than it does for most people. If you stay in the present, it's very helpful. Focus on what is happening right now.

If you should get a call from them sharing some test results, just be supportive. Don't ask a lot of questions; just let them say what's on their mind. If it's good news, express your happiness. If it's bad news, remain positive–"What can I do," or, "I'm here if you need me," or say nothing. You need to be the friend, the support system—"Let's go to a movie," or, "Let's go to the ocean," or, "Let's go to the farmer's market."

It may seem like a lot of waiting and that you are just not doing enough. Imagine that you are a firefighter just sitting there waiting at the station house. The firefighter doesn't call and say, "I'm coming to fight the fire." He waits. And, eventually he gets a call and it's pretty helpful when he shows up. The time may come when you can do something to actively help your friend. You may get a call to see if you could wash the car, mow the lawn, or pick up some groceries; any one of a number of routine things. They may seem small and insignificant, but they are not. The person fighting cancer does not have the energy, time, or focus to be doing any of those activities right now. The smallest things can bring so much relief. Stay focused on the task that is requested and just be matter of fact about it. It's not always easy to ask for help, so just show up, do the job, ask if you can help with anything while you're there, and tell them you'll see them later.

The cancer survivor may be going through chemotherapy or radiation and needs transportation. If you have been asked to drive someone to radiation or chemotherapy, your job is now that of a chauffeur. You'll note that a chauffeur does not engage the person whom they are driving in conversation, as a rule. The chauffeur stays focused on matter-of-fact questions pertaining to getting one there and back again. It's very natural to think that uplifting banter will diffuse the uncomfortable reality, but it usually produces the opposite reaction. The treatments for chemotherapy and radiation are difficult and cumulative. As one progresses in their treatment less and less energy is available and one feels the toxic or physical effects more and more. The person will likely have their defenses down, they may be depressed, they likely won't feel very good, and they very likely won't want to talk about the experience. They just want to get to the appointment and back home again to sleep.

Whatever you do, on the way home don't ask, "How was it?" It was miserable! What am I supposed to say to you? Just be a worker bee. It's not that you can't talk to them, but try to just respond to what they want to talk about or do. For me, I couldn't wait for my extra-thin milk shake following every radiation session. A little reward can go a long way. "Let me know if there is something I can do," will be all that's needed.

It's possible that you may accompany someone who is waiting in an oncology clinic. These clinics are filled with around twenty to fifty people waiting for their treatments. There can be discussion between patients about their treatments or how they are feeling. You'll notice that the communication between patients is mostly uplifting and positive, and does not involve a lot of questions about what their condition is. If you are accompanying them as a caregiver, you need to be prepared to witness some unsettling things. People are at the clinic for their treatments, not for attention or pity. If for any reason you do not think that you can remain detached while accompanying someone, you should find someone else to do this. It's okay; many doctors passed out during their first observance of surgery. But you have to step up, admit that this is too hard for you, and get someone else instead. Stepping aside and getting the right person to help will be how you provide support.

The cancer survivor may at some point be in the hospital for any number of reasons. It's usually a good idea to just let them focus on getting better by leaving them alone. However, if they have indicated to you that they would like you to come and see them, be brief, be uplifting, and don't be emotional. I've been around a number of patients who had someone with them and it was very obvious that the patient did not want that person to be there. They were worried about their own situation and what would happen to them and now they were also constantly trying to see how the visitor was reacting as well. When you watch people in the healthcare community dealing with cancer, they are very matter of fact. They do not spend a lot of time on the emotional side except to stay hopeful and positive.

The treatment phase can be very difficult for the cancer survivor. You will see that the patient usually tries to look to the bright side. Help them stay in that mental place. Do not talk about anything depressing. If they bring up things that are depressing, or if they cry, let them. Crying is a way to communicate emotion. You should not interrupt this communication any more than you would interrupt their words to you. Be available for the person so they can go through the experience, but don't pile on. What they are sharing are thoughts, feelings, anxieties, or concerns that have finally bubbled to the surface where they can accept them enough to share them with you. Nothing else is required from you than to listen; and at most say, "What can I do?" The individual is looking for you to be strong for them. You don't need to be overly cheerful and happy, but you do need to be positive and present. Statements such as, "I respect the way you're dealing with this," or, "you seem to be managing this process," or, "you sound so good," are positive things that will uplift them. They start to think, "Yeah, I am handling it pretty well." The cancer survivor goes to bed at night and wakes up wondering if they are coping effectively. Statements that indicate they are doing well are tremendously helpful.

Don't forget that to remain a strong source of support you need to take care of yourself. Eat right, get exercise, and get assistance as you need it from support groups or a counselor to help you deal with your emotions and mental attitude.

Things Not to Say to Someone Dealing with Cancer

- I read this on WebMD ...
- I found this diet that you should be on ...
- There is a new study about ...
- How was it?
- Is it going to be difficult?
- I want to be with you, keep you company, spend time with you in the hospital.
- I know someone this happened to and it didn't go well.
- What is the diagnosis?
- How much time do you have?

Positive Things to Say to Someone Dealing with Cancer

- I admire how you are handling things.

- I respect the way you are managing . . .

- If there is something I can do, let me know.

- You look really great.

- If there is something that you would like, please tell me.

Some Thoughts for the Medical Community from the Patient's Point of View

Although those of you who treat cancer and work with cancer patients, no matter what your role—oncologist, surgeon, nurse, radiation therapist, or receptionist, are dedicated people, you run the risk of getting burned out or becoming numb to the people around you. Each person can become a number on a chart, not an individual. You must constantly remind yourself that one of the most important things that you can do for the patient is to stay fresh and be engaged. It may be your fortieth appointment that day, but it is the patient's first.

If you are not engaged, the message that you send is that you are not listening. When a patient has given up so much control in their life and turned much of it over to you, they need to know that their deepest concerns will be reviewed. Do not cut them off in the middle of them telling you something, "I know what you're going to say." You may know what they are going to say, but do not deny them the right to say it. It's their first experience and it is part of their healing. And you might be surprised at what you learn if you listen to completed thoughts. How a patient says something is a diagnostic tool as much as what is said. Interruption takes that information away from you. Letting them talk reinforces the fact that you are professional, that you do listen, that you do know, and that you do care. To remain fresh just be honest and caring.

When you are talking about treatment options, don't talk about how hard this is going to be to go through. Help the patient through the process by saying, "This is going to be a little longer," or, "In the beginning this is going to be a bit easier, but as we move through treatment you will be drained and it's possible to have other complications." They don't need all the technical details, but the patient does need to know the issues and how those issues will affect their life. It helps if you talk in terms of averages to set expectations. People can handle only so much reality. Deliver the truth, but in a framework that's not too grave. Keep reminding them of the goal of the treatment; it will help them get past the treatment process and focus on the purpose of the treatment.

I would like to share a few thoughts about pain. During the course of my treatment I have had a lot of cutting done on me. There were times when I needed a small procedure done that did not involve any anesthesia. It's a little more frightening when you're wide awake and they are going to cut you. I remember one time when the physician said, "We're just going to open your throat up a little bit and reposition this drain, but it's not going to hurt. With all that you've been through, this is nothing." It's probably better not to tell me that it is trivial. The anxiety around pain and the pain itself are cumulative. I know it's going to hurt, and you know it's going to hurt. Let's be honest about that. Or, on other occasions I've been told, "You're tough. You can put up with it."

I may not be so tough depending upon how I'm feeling that day, what is about to happen to me, or any other news that I may have just received prior to my arrival—a family issue, a crisis with my job, a notice from the IRS (the IRS really does not care if you have cancer). So please, don't tell people how tough they are. Do tell them you will hurt them as little as you possibly can.

Chapter Three

Hope

In April 2009 I was told I had eleven months to live. Subsequent tests contradicted that prognosis, but I had received that initial message and I had believed it. The situation seemed pretty bleak.

As a young man I was part of a special military training program. On a particular training mission on a mountain, in freezing temperatures and snow, we were given limited rations and told to survive the bitterly cold night. At one point a member of the company became exhausted and simply gave up; he lay down in the snow and said, "I just want to sleep." Our training dictated that we get this person up and keep him moving even if we had to kick him to do so. The message was: you do not give up. I think that extraordinary training is how I moved through those first few months. I just kept moving forward. I trusted my medical team, and focused on the next right thing that they wanted me to do.

I don't know that you actually have to believe that you are going to get through this. What you do have to believe is that you will get through today; that you have control over today. The denial about your situation may even work in your favor, because in denial there is also hope.

In truth, no one knows how long they have to live. As I sit here today nearly four years from the time of my initial diagnosis, in that time period two of my very close friends have died. One was from pancreatic cancer. My other very healthy friend was at a dinner party, choked on a piece of meat, and died. He did not know that it would be his last meal. No one knows; not the doctor, not the statisticians. What we do know is that we have today, and by being here today there is the promise of tomorrow.

The Most Important Tool for the Cancer Survivor

The greater your success in getting into today and being positive about this day, the greater quality of life you will have for whatever is the remainder of your life. Every doctor or caregiver will tell you that the better your frame of mind is in dealing with this disease, the better your chances are. Developing a positive attitude as a mainstay of your treatment is really essential. So when things may not seem so good, how do you do keep your spirits up?

The first step is accepting responsibility for your own mental health. This responsibility means that you have to be proactive. Now may be a good time to enlist the aid of a professional. You will be dealing with a lot of potential change in your life and working with someone who can assist you in your decision making is frequently a helpful step. A professional counselor, especially someone who is used to working with people who have cancer, can provide an objective forum for you to discuss your fears, concerns, or strategies without the burden of your need to assess their emotional response as it would with a friend or family member. Conversation with an objective professional can keep you from feeling quite so isolated. Contacting someone early and having an initial conversation with them can be helpful. It gives them a sense of where you are as you begin this journey. They can help you monitor your mental attitude as you move through the management of your illness. You may only need them periodically, but it's nice to know that they are a resource when you do need them. They can also assist you in how to develop positive thought, and positive thought leads to positive action.

Enlisting whatever help you might need to keep your spirits and hope alive is essential. Now is not the time to be proud or vain; ditch those qualities immediately. Let those who have training or life experience buoy you through these tough waters. Although it seems counter intuitive, vulnerability begets strength, and stoicism and isolation invariably lead to weakness. For whatever reason, women are much better at this than men, including me. This is strange territory for many of us, but as the saying goes, "deal with it," and then move on.

Every day you have to get up and be positive even if you have had depressing news. Sometimes it's not so easy to know if you are succeeding. Make it your job and daily mission to find something positive to focus on—a beautiful landscape, a positive life story, an inspirational message—something from which you can draw strength and get out of yourself. Despair and self pity are your enemy. As easy as it may be to embrace those thoughts, I urge you to resist them at all costs. If there is someone close to you whose judgment you trust, enlist their aid in assessing how you are doing in resisting these thoughts; "How do *you* think I'm doing?" or, "How do I appear to you?" Sometimes a little feedback can put you back on course. If you feel the clouds starting to close in, reach out to someone who can reflect positive energy back to you. Your mental well being and attitude is paramount; it will guide everything else.

A lot of things may begin to change in your life—your physical condition, schedules, energy level. If you are able to accept a shift in the routines and the level of control you have perceived to have had in your life, it makes life much easier. A sense of humor can be a truly great gift in this regard. Your mind is a powerful asset in managing your situation.

A major step you can take in maintaining a positive attitude is to avoid everyone who does not have one. These people will crush your soul. There may be individuals who just have too much sympathy. There may be individuals who have too much unhelpful advice. You may have been close to these people in the past, but for whatever reason you now do not wish their counsel (probably still their friendship, but not their counsel) so you need to change the relationship and create some distance. Negativity is a very sharp knife and cuts much deeper than people realize. If someone says something that does not sound positive to you, stop them or get away from them. You are the guardian of your own well being. This is a way that you can take control of your life, and your mental and emotional state.

The most important thing I can tell you is to do your best to keep a positive and hopeful attitude; do not lose hope.

Using Hopeful Words and Behavior to Support the Survivor

If you are someone who has been given this very personal information, you are special to the survivor. They consider you to be someone on their side, on their team. If you recognize that role and you truly embrace the responsibility, your number one job is to provide support and hope. If you don't think you can do that job for whatever reason, you should step to the sidelines. The most supportive thing you could do is to avoid taking away the hope of a cancer survivor. Think of this as creating an aura around the person and their circumstance. It is a mindset and it is transferable. Do whatever you must to get to that mindset, and stay in that positive mode—not falsely cheerful, but genuine and positive.

If you can show up as a member of the team, there are a number of things that you can do and say that create a hopeful presence. For starters you can be the mirror that reflects back the good things. The person you are trying to support is monitoring you to reflect back on how they are doing; they're likely not a good judge of how they're doing right now. So when you see them, if you say, "You look great," or, "I like the shirt," or, "I like your shoes," you are sending messages that they appear good to you. I'm not suggesting that you be disingenuous, but that you seek something positive on which to comment.

If you ask how they are doing and they respond, "this is really too hard," you might come back with, "Is there anything right now that would make it easier for you?" or, "If I did this . . . would it be helpful?" or, "Would you like to go get a cup of coffee and talk?" You could ask, "What's on your mind?" If you see a small thing that is an action that might help them feel better or even distracts them, you can suggest that it be tackled in the present perhaps with your assistance. If you focus on things that keep them moving forward, it will help them not get stuck in worry.

The more you reflect back positive messages to them, the more they will seek your ability to reflect back to them that they are okay. They may be thinking, "Well, my face is a little burned, but maybe it doesn't look as serious as I think it does. It's probably not that noticeable." If you are positive in the face of not such good stuff, it is uplifting. As they see you become uplifted, they will become uplifted. Conversely, if you are down, it will bring them down. Bring them up. Take whatever they give you and turn it into something positive.

The most hopeful behavior is being truly in the moment with the cancer survivor. Let go of thinking about, "How much time do they have left?" They have the rest of their life! Forget about the finality; focus on the time you spend together today and make it a good day. Do this in a genuine and honest way. If you are falsely cheerful, you will appear disingenuous and no longer be deemed trustworthy. It could be a long journey and you need to be in it for the long haul.

Which brings me to a very important point: You too must find ways and strategies to keep yourself positive. Take a look at your own situation and find ways to increase your level of optimism and things that you can do for yourself. It's the old oxygen mask on the plane. You have to be present and prepared yourself in order to help someone else.

When you are with the cancer survivor, think in terms of hope; be the carrier of hope. Your hopeful attitude could very well be the tipping point of their recovery.

Suggestions for How the Medical Community Can Support a Hopeful Outlook

Those of you who deal with cancer face it every day from the perspective of your daily actions and particular focus. I would like for you to see those interactions from the other side. My observation is that medical personnel have varying degrees of empathy and understanding in dealing with cancer. As a general rule, if you are directly involved in dealing with cancer—radiation therapy, or oncology, for example—your specialty has over time given you a very incredible experiential knowledge and you are circumspect in your remarks. However, if you step outside of that specialty, one frequently finds that the opposite is true. I have had an endocrinologist say, "What did you expect, you have stage IV cancer?" That's a pretty reckless thing to say. Or I've heard, "you have to be realistic in your expectations." That's pretty limiting; how many Olympic athletes received that message? Probably not a lot of them did. I believe that this is an attempt to control the situation because many of you are actually very afraid of cancer, and you are uncomfortable talking about it or admitting that you do not have a solution. If you are not good at this, stay away from talking to the patient. Turn the conversations over to those who are better equipped to handle them or develop the appropriate skills.

The comfort level of being able to talk about cancer is also important for nurses and others who provide care. The further one gets from regular dealings with cancer patients the less they understand how to talk to them, and sometimes they say some very unhelpful things. Because of a lack of specific knowledge they frequently will use general comments such as, "Well, I'd be concerned about that." In what way would you be concerned? When queried the answer often is, "Well, I don't know." If you don't have specific knowledge, you should let someone else handle the conversation. Because you hold a position in the medical team you may give the impression of having more authority than you actually possess. The patient will likely give this authority over to you and, of course, they are constantly looking for clues as to what is happening to them. Don't overstep your bounds and take on responsibility you do not possess. This is also true for EMTs, dentists, and others with whom the patient may come in contact. If you don't actually have specific information to provide regarding the treatment, don't guess or offer advice.

So what can you do to engender hope without compromising what you understand to be a reality? You can be present in today with the patient and encourage them to live life to the fullest–whatever "fullest" means to them. Days before Virginia Clinton Kelley, mother of former President Bill Clinton, died of breast cancer she attended a Barbara Streisand concert in Las Vegas. You can encourage your patients to enjoy life. You need only be the voice of reason and support.

You may not be able to make the patient's cancer go away, but your words can make it worse. What you say and how you say it does affect your patient's mental attitude. There are ways in which you can crush hope. Phrases such as, "This is a normal progression," or, "As this gets more serious these things will happen . . ." or, "You may start to experience more and more pain," are not helpful. The patient will know if they have pain and they will call you. You do not need to put into their mind what might happen.

As a patient loses energy, their strength comes from the outside; those who provide the most strength are usually the physician or caregiver. Everyone may see the final result including the patient, but they need someone else in the room to be strong for them; not someone who hits them over the head with the reality. What gets one through is the hope of *each* day. Do not do anything to dissuade that.

In many instances discussions about hospice may arise, these should still be positive and reflect hope. If the focus remains on today, you can frame the conversation in such a way that right now you feel they would get the best care with a very individualized program focusing on their daily needs which is what hospice does. My friend who died of pancreatic cancer entered hospice willingly because they told him that he would get more rest and therefore become stronger. That was his goal—to get more rest so he could go home and be stronger. In fact, many people enter hospice, get stronger and stabilized, and are then removed from the program.

With all that you do for your patients (and all of us who are treated by you know just how very much that is), don't forget to be one who engenders hope.

Chapter Four

Strategies, Resources, and Organizing the Network

Forming networks and associations, and connecting the dots comes naturally to me. I also had the benefit of being trained by IBM in the seventies (some of the best sales training in the world) and I ranked in the top 1% of their sales team. My point is that by inclination and by training I am very good at creating networks. In spite of this, my cancer diagnosis initially shut me down. What I have to say in this section is not rocket science, but a lot of what may seem obvious was very elusive in the days following my diagnosis. It was amazing to me that some of the most important and helpful information regarding strategies, treatments, and coping did not reach me. These are some of the basic strategies and resources that I have found to be most helpful.

For the Cancer Survivor—Optimizing Your Support

In chapter one I suggested that you identify one or two people to act as your spokesperson for any communication regarding your illness. These people are the cornerstone for building your network; they are trusted individuals who will follow your requests. Their role is to relieve you of the communication activity, act as a filter to preserve your energy, and act as a representative for you in the event that you cannot communicate, for example, after surgery. These individuals need to be given your instructions for what to say, when to say it, and to whom. You also need to introduce them to your network and let the others know that these individuals will be speaking on your behalf as needed.

I suggest that you choose these people carefully; you may have to go through an iteration or two in the event that someone becomes controlling and withholds information from certain individuals, or if there is a personality conflict with others on your list. Hopefully, any bickering will not involve you. If you set this up as a system and everyone knows what is happening, it is less likely that someone may feel they have been excluded. Explain that the process is to conserve your energy, and to be sure that nothing falls through the cracks where people may miss information. Ask them to direct inquiries about your health to your designated communicators and not to you. If you have a spouse, a significant other, sibling, relative, parent or child, people may default to them for information. This may be unfair to them and it fractures the messaging process. Putting your own system in place will prevent this.

It was also suggested that you create a list of the people that would need to be contacted along with how to reach them. With all that you may need to do in the early stages of your illness this may seem like busy work, but it's better to just do it once and get it done. You may have less energy at a later time. Needless to say, if you have an urgent situation, and are taken to surgery right away, you may not have this luxury. But, if you have a little time, creating this list is worth the effort. Use your address book as a checklist. If you forget people, don't worry about it. They will surface and it's very explainable that you had a lot going on at that particular time. You will be forgiven. If someone does surface later on, your spokesperson should let you know and confirm with you that the person should be added to the list. Remember the target illustration on page 34; you may want to sort the contacts into groups if you don't want all information to go out to everyone. This list is not only for the purpose of sending information out to them; it is also the beginning structure for a formal network to support you. There are people on this list who are in it for the long term; people who will help you as needed in the days to come.

As you gather this contact list, it is a good time to think about how each individual may be a support to you. Someone may have a special skill or personality that suggests potential assistance down the road. Make a note of these details for your designated communicators. For example, you may have a neighbor (or neighbors) who could easily mow your lawn along with theirs.

You also need to clear the decks. This is the time to put all your physical, mental, and emotional focus on what needs to be done to fight your illness. Anything that can be put aside should be, at least for the time being—little league games, weddings, anything that is a potential drain on you. There may be a big project that you are involved with at work; think about who most understands what you are bringing to the table and could represent you for a while when you are in a treatment stage. If something is so important in your life that you cannot let it go, common sense will dictate that, but depending upon your diagnosis most things need to take second place to your treatment. I had the opportunity to attend a very prestigious event in New York where I was to be recognized and receive an award. I was worried about another surgery and I was afraid I would lose my voice. As much as I wanted to go, the event was just not right for me at that time. If something doesn't feel right, don't do it. A gift of this process is finding out what is really important to you.

All through your life financial planners, attorneys, and insurance agents have advised you to have your affairs in order. Your affairs likely are in some stage of readiness, but don't be embarrassed if they're not. It is really important for you to focus on the most important elements of this task as soon as possible. It may have been a while since you reviewed documents and there may be items that are out of date or no longer reflect the same intention that you had when they were first prepared. Recently, an acquaintance of mine went in for a checkup and they discovered a serious issue with lung cancer; he was sent to radiation therapy right away. In the hospital talking with a mutual friend he expressed concern about his estate; he had a daughter by a first marriage and step children by a second marriage which did not last very long. He wanted his biological daughter to inherit his estate. They were going to get an attorney, prepare documents representing his intentions, have him review it, and then get a notary public to witness the signing. I urged them to call the attorney imme-diately, and along with a notary public have them meet with him at the hospital so that he could declare his wishes, and have it signed and notarized on the spot. I was pretty sure that if they explained to him why they were doing it this way—just to be sure his daughter was protected as he wished—that he would be fine with it. He signed the documents in his hospi-tal room the same day. Two days later he slipped into a coma and never came out it. He died two weeks later. This exam-ple is not to scare you; it's an unlikely scenario. However, it should point out that we do not know when things in our life may change or that we may not have warning about those changes. It's a good idea to do this preparation to ensure that your affairs will be handled as you wish them to be should something happen to you.

The other major document that you need to prepare is an advanced health directive. In the absence of expressing your wishes for your care, others will decide for you. No one knows when that may be an issue, but you know that you may be going through procedures that carry some risks of complica-tion. It only makes sense to take the time to plan while you are clear.

At one time I was dealing with a family whose mother was quite ill and was slipping in and out of a coma. She had significant financial resources but had never created a trust or a will. Her family needed more money for her care, but they were not able to access the funds because no one had been given power of attorney. She died. We never know when we may walk around the corner and be hit by a bus. It is a reality that a time may come when you are not as mentally clear as you are now—coma, dementia, medication, or pain. If you don't need these documents, it doesn't matter; if you do need them, they are in place. Be sure you have designated a power of attorney for your financial affairs and a power of attorney for your health directives.

There are other details that you would be wise to consider while you're doing planning. It will be a road map for those who may need to help you. Think through scenarios for your pets, your property, your car; not only their possible disposition, but what maintenance would they need if you are incapacitated for a period of time. It's just good planning.

One of the surprises that I encountered in my early attempts to understand my new situation turned out to be that my greatest form of outside support was never presented to me. I found it accidentally. I want you to have it available from the beginning. As soon as you have a diagnosis identifying a specific type of cancer, locate the support group for your specific cancer—support groups exist for every type of cancer.

You will probably be directed, as I was, by your physician or the hospital to the cancer support group operated by the hospital. The primary task of any hospital will be to deal with your medical treatment. All of the options for additional support that can help you are usually not something that they monitor. The search for complementary support is left to the patient and friends and family to sort out. The hospital support group is a diverse group of people with different types of cancer in varying stages. Other than the fact that they all have cancer they usually have very little in common.

I had thyroid cancer which is statistically not a very prevalent form of cancer. I was quite interested in this type of cancer because it was the one that I had. I stumbled upon THYCA (Thyroid Cancer Survivors Association), a support group focused specifically on my type of cancer. These people were like me. They had similar treatments, issues, and doctors. After I contacted them they wanted all the details of my situation and had opinions on everything (but unlike my caring friends who were offering advice these people had been through similar experiences). It was so refreshing because I no longer felt like I was in the foxhole alone. They offered local information about which doctors had the most success and about things which were not working quite so well. You will find tremendous support for your situation in this group, and everyone will be familiar with what may lay ahead for you. They are also up on the latest trials and techniques, and the locations which are most successful in treating your cancer. I urge you to get in touch with these people as soon as possible.

Do an internet search for your type of cancer—breast, lung, brain—and "support group." The national group usually has a hotline that is not manned twenty-four hours a day, but will usually return a call the next day. They'll give you the names of other cancer survivors whom you can talk to, and they are very empathetic and understanding. They usually have books, pamphlets, and other support materials. This will give you information to use in discussion with your own medical team.

There are also usually local support groups who meet monthly. They know everything you need to know about the local care community—which doctors are performing the most surgeries for your specific area and who is having the greatest success. They will have doctors and researchers dealing with your type of cancer as guests who will talk about the newest information or experiences, and they will stay around and answer your specific questions. These doctors love this type of event; they are talking to those in the wheel house of what they do, but they also hear or learn things that can give them a new direction. This is a really valuable opportunity for you; it's outside information and advice independent of the particular institutions with which you are associated. It's another way to advocate for you.

There are also the national cancer associations—the American Cancer Society, and the National Cancer Institute—which can provide a lot of helpful information in specific areas. They offer information on staying healthy during treatment recovery, handling financial matters, and managing cancer treatments.

The Most Important Things for the Cancer Survivor to Do

- Create a personal supportive network.

- Locate the support group that focuses on your specific type of cancer.

- Appoint a power of attorney for your financial affairs and power of attorney for your health directives.

- Never lose hope.

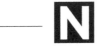

What Friends and Family Can Do to Be Supportive

If the survivor that you are supporting has identified someone as a communication traffic controller, use the system that they have put in place. If the cancer survivor has not done this, carefully follow their lead for how they want to receive communication. Just be aware that any interaction may be a drain on their energy and do what you can to preserve it. So, what can you do proactively to be supportive?

Depending upon where the individual is in their treatment, a number of opportunities may surface. These small routine things will definitely be helpful—more than you can imagine, and being helpful will likely make you feel better as well. If you have special talents or skills, make them known. You may have time slots available to do whatever is needed; share that availability. Don't be offended if you aren't called to do something, remember it's the time and energy management here that is most supportive. But having people in the wings is really important as well, physically and emotionally. The support of the people around you is important—even if they just stand and wait. There is strength in numbers.

When a need emerges the individuals who are managing the communication flow can either post a task where some help would be appreciated, or they may refer to a list of people who have already volunteered for specific activities. It's amazing how draining the most routine activities can be when you are fighting cancer: You go to pick up the dry cleaning and it isn't ready, or there is an excessively long line at the bank when you're already too tired to stand. These daily activities can be just too much, so if someone can shuttle children back and forth to activities, mow the lawn, clean the car, pick up groceries, or clear out the gutters, it is a genuine relief to the survivor. Whether or not you are the one who receives a call, this is not about your relationship with the person (or anybody else's relationship with them); it's only about building a supportive collective. Sometimes you get called, sometimes someone else gets called.

In the event that you are geographically close to a number of the people on the cancer survivor's list, you might want to find out who else is on the list and form your own local support group. By getting together you can express your own feelings, fears, and anxieties in a place where others understand and share what you are going through. Have a monthly potluck at someone's home; it's a social way to share information and help uplift your spirit. You'll come up with your own great ideas to provide support for the cancer survivor and for each other.

Some people do not do well in groups. Some people simply prefer to discuss their private thoughts in a one-on-one situation. There is nothing wrong with this way of communicating, it is simply a preference. If you learn of a personal support group, and do not want to attend events, it does not indicate a lack of support for this person. You may end up with a strong, personal relationship with someone else on the patient's list, and you can support each other in that way.

If the cancer survivor has not designated a communicator, you can use a local personal group to provide task relief. List what would be helpful and work out a schedule to be sure everything gets covered. The only caveat is that you don't rely on the person who is ill to help manage the schedule. Keep them informed of how it's being handled, but just show up and perform the task. Remember it's about the conservation of time and energy.

Individuals diagnosed with cancer are not always feeling horrible. It's important to know that, too. The treatment stage can be rough (although not for everyone). But when they are not in a treatment phase, they may feel quite like their old self. Frequently though, no one else will see them that way. I've said that cancer carries a stigma; it's not like a heart attack, or a broken leg, or a car accident. Those are things that all of us can understand. Cancer is difficult to understand; it is actually hundreds of different diseases with the common feature that it's hard to predict where things will go, and so there is a lot of fear. Because of that fear people don't want to talk about it. In that dance of fear and concern, they frequently act uncharacteristically. The most common outcome is to just stay away. For the person with cancer this becomes very isolating. They already feel like they're in a different class and they are seeking some normalcy in their life, some relief from thinking about cancer. If you are supporting someone with cancer, you need to be aware of the feelings of being singled out and isolated. I know that I keep saying let them be, don't drain their energy, don't bother them. But that refers to talking about their disease and transferring your own emotions on to them.

So, what can you do to contribute some normalcy in their life? Keep inviting them to dinner or to events. They may decline a particular invitation, but that doesn't mean they will not accept the next one. When they do show up, you may see a decline in their physical condition; okay, it is what it is. Focus on what is positive without discussing their illness, "It's great to see you." Don't let the illness be the elephant in the room. It's a balance of protection and outreach which is very individual, and the best that you can do is to be aware of it.

I was discussing my intentions to write this book with one of my oncologists and she really supported the effort. In the sixties her father was diagnosed with cancer. She recounted that one of her worst memories was when they were invited to a dinner party with friends. At his place setting (and only his place setting) were a paper plate and plastic utensils. We've come pretty far since then, but the individual still does not want to be the focus of attention. They want to blend in like everyone else. They deal with cancer twenty-four hours a day and this is an opportunity for them to step away from it. They are getting out having a good time like anyone else.

Cancer changes the relationship with food. Food is one of the ways in which societal groups comfort themselves and each other. The most natural thing in the world is to offer food as a form of support. If this offer of food is for the family of a cancer survivor to free up their time in other areas that is fine. But to a person battling cancer, food may take on a different reality; palates change and the ability to eat a certain food changes. You may specially prepare and offer the cookies that have been their favorite holiday tradition and get a simple, "no, thank you," and that may deflate you a bit. Palates change a lot with treatments for cancer. With chemotherapy, foods that you previously would never have consumed are now your favorite thing. The foods you always gravitated to for comfort may now be completely unpalatable.

For me, my relationship to food changed most dramatically with radiation. On one hand, I pretty much lost my sense of taste. All of a sudden I started drinking coffee which I hadn't had in fifteen years; because at this point it was the only thing I could taste. On the other hand, I was getting burned every day and just like a burn after you have touched the stove, you don't want to put things on it that hurt. I found that any spicy food or anything with acidity was painful, such as one of my favorite foods–lasagna. One unfortuante day I made the mistake of brushing my teeth and then using Listerine– ouch! I found a new love for Jell-O in any color, and thin milkshakes. Chemotherapy, radiation, medications can all alter the taste buds. There are also potential airway issues and choking hazards.

The most supportive thing that you can do is to always ask what the cancer patient would like in a matter-of-fact way (calling attention to their food choices in public can be embarrassing for many people). Do not make assumptions about what you think they may want or need. Do not make comments on what may appear to you to be a rather odd combination of foods. Put on a coat of armor for yourself and do not take any rejection of food personally. Most of these changes are not permanent and what works one day may change completely the next day.

There may come a time when the person is in the hospital. Hospitals are not very restful places; there is a lot of activity—people talking in the halls, nurses poking you for one reason or another all night long. For someone who is already worn out, the energy needed to try and have a simple conversation may be just too much. Resist the desire to go and see them (yes, I know that you want to verify for yourself that they are okay). Send flowers if you think that would be uplifting for them, or make a donation to the cancer support group in their name. Send a card.

If you get a request from them to visit, by all means go but stay focused on being positive and be aware of their energy level. They may not be in much pain because of their medication, but they'll surely be tired. Depending upon the type of cancer that the person has there may be some hard things to deal with emotionally. There are a lot of difficult physical things around cancer. If you do visit you need to be prepared for this, and if you think you cannot be in the room without losing control you should stay home. Do not burst into their room in tears or reflect your sadness. You need to be able to walk into the room remaining positive, upbeat, and hopeful.

Remember you are their mirror; they may not know what they look like and may be very fearful about what that is. Your smiling face and comments such as, "I like your room," or, "You look great," or, I'm surprised you're up and moving about so well," have the ability to reset their attitude. I don't know anybody who doesn't want to be told they look good. If they've lost their hair, you could say "I like your scarf," or "I like your eye shadow."

People are often at a loss for words when they first walk in so talk about the room, the flowers, the TV, how great everything looks, how clean the room is, how many people are around to help them, and how friendly they are. You can talk about mutual interests or sports. Light joking is always helpful. If the person doesn't feel so good, they may think, "Well, at least I'm in a nice place." If they come back with a comment such as, "things aren't that great," respond with something like, "You're very brave. You're doing incredibly well under difficult circumstances, I don't know if I could do that." Continually reflecting the positive will have impact.

**Phrases to Have at the Ready When Visiting
Someone in the Hospital**

- You look great.

- You seem to be bouncing back quickly.

- You have great color.

- You seem alert.

- I like your room.

- Your room seems very comfortable.

- Everyone is so friendly.

There are also resources for *you* that will help you remain strong. The same specific cancer support group that your friend or family member uses to guide them has information available for you as well. In addition, national organizations such as the American Cancer Society or the National Cancer Institute have a wealth of information for caregivers and those supporting someone with cancer. They have booklets specifically for caregivers and how to cope emotionally or guides for teenagers dealing with a sibling or a parent with cancer. Your greatest support, however, may come from those who share a connection with the person you are supporting.

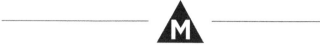

A Few More Thoughts for the Medical Team

You all know a lot about cancer and working with people who have cancer. What you do not know is the unique life experience of each patient. It's just possible they may have some ideas on how best to manage their situation. While you suggest strategies or resources based upon your experience, the patient may know that other options will simply be a better choice for them. They may also come up with some new ways to manage things. They need the support system that they can put together for themselves. Don't be offended if they do not choose your path for seeking outside support. They may try their own way and then come back to yours, but they must do what feels right for them.

I was part of a focus group run by a group of surgeons and the question was asked, "Does anyone have trouble swallowing?" Now, I'm sitting in a group of people who have all had throat surgery; "yeah!" was the response. I had had the good fortune to be taught how to swallow by a speech pathologist and because the lesson was counter intuitive I thought I would share it. I volunteered the information, which is that you first grit your teeth and then swallow. The surgeons said, "You're kidding me. No, that makes sense." This was new information for them that they could share with future patients. If you really pay attention, your patients can teach you a lot about their disease which will help you in your practice.

Chapter Five

Special Situations

At the time I was diagnosed with cancer, I had been in alcohol dependency recovery for over thirty years. I no longer attended a formal support group on any regular basis, but following my diagnosis, one of the first things that I did was to find a local group and begin to once again attend regularly. My long history of dealing with individuals with a dependency indicated that having cancer might put me at risk emotionally. I was acutely aware that I needed a close-knit support group that focused on my well being, one that understood me personally. In an effort to protect myself, I inadvertently discovered one of my greatest sources of unconditional support as I worked through my illness.

I am fortunate that my life experience has led me down this path, but many individuals are less experienced. As I have sat in the oncology waiting room, in support group sessions, or focus groups with other cancer patients, I've been able to learn a great deal from their situations. I have observed that individuals in a number of particular circumstances may need a special type of conversation, and may need additional kinds of support. These areas are less about, "what not to say," and more about "you really need to talk about this."

Alcohol, Drugs, and Prescription Medications

It is essential that if an individual is affected by alcohol, drugs, or prescription medications in any way, they must be completely honest with their medical team. A person may not even have accepted that they have a dependency, but it is critical that the medical team understands the reality of the situation. Denial is the hallmark of dependency, but in this case, the consequence can actually be life or death.

The treatment of any cancer is usually a very complicated formula. The last thing that the medical team needs is an unknown that they did not factor in and cannot identify. For example, if an individual has become a maintenance drinker, at some point crossing over the line from casual drinking, they may not have noticed the change and may not tell the medical team. This person is then admitted to the hospital, no longer has access to alcohol, and while they are on the operating table they go into the DTs (*delirium tremens* is severe shaking which can occur in an acute episode of alcohol withdrawal). The surgeon is doing delicate work and has no idea what is going on. Or the individual comes out of surgery and is now on some pretty strong medication, and then goes into the DTs. The medical team may think the symptoms are a reaction to the medication and the individual may not be able to communicate at that time to inform the situation. The same is true of drugs; if you are still using them you could end up with a wicked drug interaction. The hospital may not pick up these substances in the lab work.

If an individual is receiving treatments for chemotherapy or radiation and they are self-medicating, they are messing up the delicate formula that is designed to cure them. I can't imagine anyone consuming alcohol while receiving radiation therapy on the throat or mouth; it would just hurt too much. There are also side effects to these substances that work against one's emotional health—many are depressants.

Family members may not be aware of any substance abuse issues, so it is up to the cancer patient to truly come clean about their situation. If an individual is concerned about where they are on the alcohol spectrum, they can stop consuming it for several days and see how they feel. It's probably better to err on the side of caution so nothing is lost in contacting a dependency support group and talking with someone. These groups are anonymous—no one wants to know about you, they only want to help. At the very least, letting the medical team know that there may be an issue is important.

There is another potential consequence for those who have been in recovery from alcohol or drug dependencies—relapse. Cancer creates a pretty stressful mental environment and it can trigger a relapse for some people. A positive, proactive step for someone who falls into this situation would be to reach out to a dependency support group. It would have the immediate effect of stabilizing behaviors, but may also serve as a wonderful additional system of support throughout the illness—one that is not about cancer.

If you think any of these situations describes you, let your medical team know. To *not* talk about your specific issue is a recipe for disaster; you cannot afford it.

Depression and Suicide

For someone fighting cancer to be depressed and have thoughts of suicide is not unusual. As an individual moves through surgeries and treatments they cycle through pain, nausea, and exhaustion which is generally followed by recovery and feeling better. When one is in a great deal of pain or heavily medicated and cannot envision that state changing, and when one is left alone a lot, it is not uncommon for that person to contemplate suicide. Sometimes the fear of what's ahead may trigger these thoughts. Sometimes it is the loss of one's past life. If you think of these thoughts as a library and walk through to occasionally take a look at them, I would not be concerned. But if you find that you want to stay in the room or if it seems like a viable plan, you should talk to someone about it. Sometimes you are so sick that you cannot imagine ever feeling better; but you very well may begin to feel better through the course of treatment. These thoughts are an indicator that you are not in a good place. I'm not making any moral judgment here as to right or wrong, I'm only suggesting that it is not a good state to be in alone and I suggest that you talk to someone. I have been sick enough and in enough pain that these thoughts came into my mind. They didn't stay, but I was amazed at how real they were.

Palliative Care and Hospice

The discussions about palliative care and hospice are different for every individual. When one has exhausted curative options, the discussion shifts to one of comfort and quality of life. The medical team will determine when it is the right time to have these discussions. These conversations are often not disclosed or shared with others—even the people closest to them. You may be the caregiver for someone with dementia or the parent of a child with cancer—individuals who cannot advocate for themselves—in which case you will be having these discussions. The issue at hand is quality of life.

Palliative care is specialized care for managing symptoms during an acute health issue or during curative treatment. Many individuals choose to enter a palliative care program to receive the benefits offered by symptom management experts. This type of care focuses on managing pain and other symptoms to provide comfort. One can be in palliative care for a very lengthy period and anyone can qualify.

Hospice is a type of care that focuses on the daily needs and desires of those deemed to be in the end stage of life, and it includes support for those closest to the patient. One may enter hospice and then become stabilized enough to leave it. Hospice care is very special care; the focus of hospice is to address clearly the physical, emotional, and spiritual needs of an individual. They frequently use complementary therapies such as aromatherapy or music therapy to make one comfortable. They can also help fulfill final wishes.

There is a point at which one may say, "No more." My mother did after she had surgery to remove colon polyps. She said, "I don't ever want to do that again." We respected her wishes; it was her choice. It is all about quality of life. There is only one person who can make these choices—the individual, or in some limited circumstances their representative.

Chapter Six

The Rest of Your Life

From sitting in numerous ear, nose, and throat, and head and neck clinics, it's easy for me to divide the room into those who have given up and those who have not. My own opinion is that you have the rest of your life to live, whatever that is. No doctor can tell you how long that is and they are certainly not able to determine the quality of your life. I've seen people lead remarkable lives in great pain. Others have had little pain, but have had the sword of Damocles hanging over their head. I believe that if you have a positive attitude, surround yourself with positive people, read positive things, and do positive things, it can only make your quality of life better. You only have a few choices about attitude when you get here; I choose to make the best of it.

Now there are some other things that you can do if you have been diagnosed with cancer to improve your circumstance: Believe it or not, just like your mother told you, eat green, orange, and red vegetables every day along with some healthy protein. Go to farmer's markets and make a game of finding healthy new things. Bring them home and cook them. My triumph is that I learned to cook spinach—by myself! Make it a journey on behalf of your well being—physical and mental. I guarantee that you'll feel better.

I know that I've said this before, but no matter what type of cancer you have, a specific support group exists. Use them. They are people in the same circumstances that you are. You'll have a lot in common right away and you will make new friends. Get around the people who have been successful at this and who will gladly give you their support and hope.

Do things that keep your spirits up. Some people like to do a daily journal; they find it clarifies their thoughts. If you like to go to the racetrack, go to the racetrack. If there is an activity that you like, do it—I like to play golf. Play golf, just don't keep score. If the ball gets stuck under the tree, kick it out; the U.S. Open is safe. Do the stuff that you enjoy with people who are living life. Because that is what you are doing, you are living life.

A Few Words to Friends and Family

It is my hope that this book will provide you with insight into what lies behind your conversations with a cancer survivor, and why they may react in a particular way. Take the phrases that are meaningful to you and practice them so that they become an automatic response that is reassuring.

An offshoot of learning what to say is likely to be that you recall other times when you did not say the most appropriate things. A friend recalled the time that her sister was diagnosed with several melanoma lesions on her back. They had been removed and all looked well. It was at that point that my friend found out about them. Thinking that everything was okay now, she thought it best to take the high road and be light about what seemed to be a near miss. What one doesn't know (unless you have been diagnosed yourself) is that with cancer, there are always footsteps. If everything is completely okay, why do you have to go for regular checkups? Even those who have been in remission for decades will tell you, they are always looking over their shoulder. My friend's sister was, I believe, probably hurt that her condition wasn't taken seriously enough by my friend. And my friend realized that she said what she thought would make her sister feel better without understanding any of the feelings her sister was having. But just as my friend cannot take back what she said, you also cannot take back past remarks—but you can learn from them. You can now begin with, "I'm sorry. What can I do?" You can just be there.

❧

In January of this year, seventy-three-year-old actress Valerie Harper was diagnosed with a rare form of brain cancer. In interviews on CBS *This Morning* and *The Doctors*, she shared a message to the world, "I'm living in the moment. Don't go to the funeral until the day of the funeral. While you're living—live."

There is an old proverb: "We can't control the wind, we can adjust our sails." I wish you all smooth sailing.

About the Author

Paul Bishop has spent decades in high-end sales in both the technology and finance industries. His prescient whistleblower complaint in early 2006 was featured in an Emmy award-winning *60 Minutes* segment—"World of Trouble."

Two months after the segment aired Paul was diagnosed with stage IV thyroid cancer. He offers this guide for the person who has been diagnosed with cancer, their friends and family, and the medical community in order to create a more effective way to build support.

Lightning Source UK Ltd.
Milton Keynes UK
UKOW06n0723150616

276296UK00001BA/2/P